# DAPOXETINE GUIDE

# A Comprehensive Resource for Men's Sexual Health and Thriving Intimacy

## Dr. Gideon Robert

## Table of Contents

- CHAPTER ONE ........................................ 4
  - What is Dapoxetine? ...................... 4
- CHAPTER TWO ....................................... 7
  - Mechanism of action and applications ...................................... 7
- CHAPTER THREE ................................. 11
  - How Does Dapoxetine Work? .. 11
- CHAPTER FOUR .................................. 14
  - How is Dapoxetine generally administered? ............................... 14
- CHAPTER FIVE ..................................... 18
  - What are the potential benefits of using Dapoxetine? ................... 18
- CHAPTER SIX ........................................ 22
  - Contraindications: ...................... 22
- CHAPTER SEVEN ................................. 27

Drug Interactions...........................27

CHAPTER EIGHT..............................32

What are the common side effects of Dapoxetine?...............32

CHAPTER NINE................................38

Key Takeaways regarding Dapoxetine....................................38

THE END ...........................................43

# CHAPTER ONE

## What is Dapoxetine?

Dapoxetine is a short-acting selective serotonin reuptake inhibitor (SSRI) that is primarily used to treat premature ejaculation in men. PE is a common sexual disorder characterized by early ejaculation and little sexual arousal, which frequently causes distress and interpersonal difficulties.

Dapoxetine works by boosting serotonin levels in the nerve system, hence delaying ejaculation. Unlike other SSRIs used to treat depression and anxiety, which take weeks to work, dapoxetine's effects are immediate, usually within 1-3 hours of oral administration. Because of its fast action, it is ideal for use before to sexual activity.

The average dapoxetine dosage is 30 mg to 60 mg, administered 1-3 hours before sexual intercourse. Its short half-life of roughly 1.5 hours lessens the risk of long-term negative effects and the likelihood of drug buildup in the body. This feature sets dapoxetine apart from other SSRIs used to treat mood disorders, which require regular daily dose and have longer half-lives.

Dapoxetine has been shown in clinical investigations to improve ejaculation control and latency time. It has also been demonstrated to increase sexual satisfaction while reducing the psychological burden of PE on men and their partners. Common adverse effects include nausea, dizziness, headaches, and diarrhea, which are usually minor and temporary.

Dapoxetine is not recommended for males who have cardiac problems, have significant liver impairment, or are taking certain medications, such as monoamine oxidase inhibitors (MAOIs) or other serotonergic pharmaceuticals, because of the risk of serotonin syndrome.

Dapoxetine, which has been approved in various countries, is an effective, well-tolerated therapy choice for men suffering from PE that can significantly enhance their quality of life and sexual health.

## CHAPTER TWO

### Mechanism of action and applications

Dapoxetine's method of action is as a selective serotonin reuptake inhibitor. Dapoxetine increases the availability of serotonin in the nervous system by decreasing its reuptake in the synaptic cleft. This increase in serotonin levels boosts the neurotransmitter's action in the brain, particularly in regions that control ejaculation. The enhanced serotonin activity slows the ejaculatory reflex, lengthening the time to ejaculation and enhancing control over the process.

Unlike standard SSRIs used to treat depression and anxiety, which take several weeks to produce therapeutic effects, dapoxetine's effects appear within 1-3 hours of oral administration. This allows for on-demand use before to sexual activity, rather than constant daily dose.

Dapoxetine is primarily used to treat premature ejaculation (PE) in men. PE is characterized as early ejaculation with low sexual arousal, which can cause emotional distress and interpersonal problems. Dapoxetine helps reduce PE symptoms by delaying ejaculation, increasing sexual satisfaction and lowering the psychological burden associated with the illness.

The average dapoxetine dosage is 30 mg to 60 mg, administered 1-3 hours before sexual intercourse. Its short half-life of roughly 1.5 hours lessens the likelihood of long-term side effects and the possibility of drug buildup, setting it apart from other SSRIs with longer half-lives used to treat mood disorders.

Clinical investigations have shown that dapoxetine increases intravaginal ejaculatory latency time (IELT) and improves ejaculatory control. Common adverse effects include nausea, dizziness, headaches, and diarrhea, which are usually minor and temporary.

Dapoxetine is not recommended for men with certain medical conditions or those taking specified drugs due to the possibility of unpleasant reactions such as serotonin syndrome. Dapoxetine, which has been approved in multiple countries, is an effective and well-tolerated treatment option for men with PE that can significantly improve their quality of life and sexual health.

# CHAPTER THREE

## How Does Dapoxetine Work?

Dapoxetine is a selective serotonin reuptake inhibitor (SSRI) that was developed primarily to treat men's premature ejaculation (PE). Its mode of action is based on the manipulation of serotonin levels in the brain, which play an important role in the ejaculatory process.

Serotonin is a neurotransmitter that regulates many brain activities, including mood, sleep, and sexual behavior. Serotonin regulates the timing of the ejaculatory reflex. Dapoxetine inhibits serotonin reuptake, increasing its availability in the synaptic cleft and thereby improving serotonergic activity.

Dapoxetine is readily absorbed after consumption, reaching peak plasma concentrations within 1-3 hours. Because of its rapid beginning of effect, it can be used as needed rather than every day. The enhanced serotonin activity in the synaptic cleft enhances the inhibition of the ejaculatory reflex, resulting in a delayed ejaculation.

Dapoxetine's principal site of action is the lateral paragigantocellular nucleus (LPGi) in the brainstem, which is an important region for controlling ejaculation. Dapoxetine efficiently delays the transmission of ejaculatory signals by increasing serotonin levels in this location, hence increasing the intravaginal ejaculatory latency time (IELT).

Dapoxetine's short half-life of around 1.5 hours ensures that it acts fast and is promptly cleared from the body, lowering the risk of long-term side effects and systemic buildup. This pharmacokinetic profile is useful for treating PE since it is consistent with the episodic nature of sexual activity.

Dapoxetine has been demonstrated in clinical trials to considerably improve ejaculation control, raise IELT, and improve overall sexual pleasure in both men and their partners. Its most common side effects include nausea, dizziness, headache, and diarrhea, which are usually minor and temporary.

Overall, dapoxetine's specific impact on serotonin reuptake, combined with its favorable pharmacokinetic features, make it an effective and well-tolerated therapy option for men who experience premature ejaculation.

## CHAPTER FOUR

### How is Dapoxetine generally administered?

Dapoxetine is normally taken orally in tablet form. The normal dosage is 30 mg to 60 mg, taken 1-3 hours before sexual activity. This timing enables dapoxetine to reach peak plasma concentrations and exhibit its effects when needed. The drug's fast onset of action makes it suitable for treating premature ejaculation (PE), as it enables on-demand management rather than requiring continual daily administration.

Before beginning dapoxetine treatment, a complete medical evaluation is required to ensure that the patient has no contraindications, such as substantial heart issues, severe liver damage, or interactions with other drugs. Once cleared, the initial dose is usually 30 mg. Depending on the patient's response and tolerance, the dose can be increased to 60 mg. To avoid potentially harmful side effects such as esophageal discomfort, consume the pills whole with a full glass of water.

Dapoxetine has a short half-life of about 1.5 hours, thus it is quickly cleared from the body, lowering the chance of long-term side effects or drug accumulation. This feature makes it appropriate for use soon before sexual activity, which corresponds to the episodic nature of PE.

Patients should avoid drinking alcohol while taking dapoxetine since it can increase some of its side effects, such as dizziness and drowsiness. Patients should also be mindful of potential interactions with other drugs, especially those that impact the central nervous system or are processed by the liver.

Common dapoxetine adverse effects include nausea, headache, dizziness, and diarrhea, which are usually minor and temporary. If side effects persist or become problematic, patients should visit their physician about possible dose modifications or other treatments.

Regular follow-up appointments are recommended to assess the treatment's effectiveness and address any concerns or side effects. Following these instructions, dapoxetine can be efficiently administered to treat premature ejaculation, enhancing sexual pleasure and overall quality of life for those affected.

## CHAPTER FIVE

### What are the potential benefits of using Dapoxetine?

The potential benefits of utilizing dapoxetine to treat premature ejaculation (PE) are numerous and important, enhancing both sexual function and general quality of life for those affected. Here are several significant advantages:

Improved Control of Ejaculation:

Dapoxetine significantly delays ejaculation by increasing serotonergic activity in the brain, namely in areas that control the ejaculatory reflex. This leads to greater control over ejaculation and a longer intravaginal ejaculatory delay time.

Increased sexual satisfaction:

Dapoxetine improves men's sexual experience by delaying ejaculation. This not only benefits the individual, but also increases their partner's sexual satisfaction, thereby boosting the overall quality of the sexual relationship.

Rapid onset of action:

Unlike other SSRIs, which might take weeks to produce results, dapoxetine works within 1-3 hours of ingestion. Because of its quick onset, it is ideal for on-demand use, allowing men to take the medicine just before sexual activity.

Flexible dosing:

Dapoxetine is available in 30 mg and 60 mg dosages, allowing for individualized dosing based on response and tolerance. This adaptability helps to improve treatment outcomes and manage any negative effects.

Reduced psychological distress:

PE can cause severe psychological suffering, including feelings of shame, irritation, and anxiety. Dapoxetine can reduce negative feelings by improving ejaculation control, hence improving general mental well-being.

Well-tolerated, with manageable side effects.

Dapoxetine's adverse effects, which include nausea, headache, dizziness, and diarrhea, are often minor and temporary. Its short half-life minimizes the possibility of long-term negative effects and drug buildup in the body.

Improved Relationship Satisfaction:

By treating the issue of PE, dapoxetine can improve relationship satisfaction while minimizing stress and tension connected to sexual performance concerns.

Quality of Life Improvement:

Overall, dapoxetine can help men with PE improve their quality of life by restoring sexual confidence and strengthening romantic relationships.

# CHAPTER SIX

## Contraindications:

Dapoxetine is contraindicated in certain medical conditions and scenarios due to potential dangers and side effects. Here are the main contraindications for dapoxetine:

Cardiovascular Conditions:

Men with severe heart failure, conduction problems (e.g., heart block), or a history of myocardial infarction should avoid taking dapoxetine. The medicine has the potential to produce orthostatic hypotension and syncope, which can be dangerous for patients with compromised cardiovascular health.

Liver impairment:

Dapoxetine is metabolized in the liver and is therefore contraindicated in persons with moderate to severe hepatic impairment. Liver impairment can cause higher medication levels and an increased risk of side effects.

Concomitant use with specific medications:

Dapoxetine should not be combined with monoamine oxidase inhibitors (MAOIs) since it increases the risk of serotonin syndrome, which can be fatal. A washout time of at least 14 days is recommended between discontinuing MAOIs and initiating dapoxetine.

It is also contraindicated in combination with other SSRIs, serotonin-norepinephrine reuptake inhibitors (SNRIs), tricyclic antidepressants, and certain antipsychotics due to an increased risk of serotonin syndrome.

Potent CYP3A4 inhibitors (e.g., ketoconazole, ritonavir) should not be taken with dapoxetine because they can raise dapoxetine levels and increase the risk of adverse effects.

Neurological Conditions:

Men who have a history of mania or severe depression should avoid taking dapoxetine. The medication's serotonergic action may worsen these symptoms.

Hypersensitivity:

Individuals who have a known hypersensitivity to dapoxetine or any of its excipients should not take it since allergic reactions may occur.

Moderate to severe renal impairment:

Patients with moderate to severe renal impairment should not use dapoxetine since it may change pharmacokinetics and increase the likelihood of adverse effects.

Orthostatic hypotension:

Men who are prone to orthostatic hypotension should avoid dapoxetine since it might exacerbate the condition, resulting in dizziness, fainting, and severe harm.

Alcohol consumption:

Concurrent use of alcohol and dapoxetine is not recommended because of the increased risk of central nervous system symptoms such as dizziness, drowsiness, and poor judgment, which can increase the possibility of injury.

## CHAPTER SEVEN
### Drug Interactions

Dapoxetine may interact with a variety of drugs, resulting in potentially serious side effects or reduced efficacy. Understanding these interactions is critical to the proper use of dapoxetine. Here are some significant medication interactions:

Monoamine Oxidase Inhibitors (MAOI):

Concurrent use of dapoxetine with MAOIs is not recommended due to the danger of serotonin syndrome, a potentially fatal illness characterized by symptoms including agitation, hallucinations, rapid heart rate, and heat. When switching between these drugs, a minimum 14-day washout time is necessary.

Other Serotonergic Drugs:

Combining dapoxetine with other SSRIs, SNRIs, tricyclic

antidepressants, or other drugs that boost serotonin levels can also result in serotonin syndrome. If these medications are used together, they must be closely monitored and maybe dose adjusted.

CYP3A4 inhibitors:

Potent CYP3A4 inhibitors, including ketoconazole, itraconazole, ritonavir, and clarithromycin, can raise dapoxetine plasma levels, increasing the risk of side effects. It is not recommended to take dapoxetine along with these inhibitors.

CYP2D6 inhibitors:

Moderate to strong CYP2D6 inhibitors, such as fluoxetine, paroxetine, and quinidine, might also increase dapoxetine levels, necessitating caution and potential dose modifications.

Phosphodiesterase Type 5 (PDE5) Inhibitors:

Co-administration of PDE5 inhibitors such as sildenafil (Viagra), tadalafil (Cialis), and vardenafil (Levitra) may raise the risk of orthostatic hypotension and syncope. When taking both drugs simultaneously, patients should be kept on guard for potential side effects.

Thioridazine:

Dapoxetine should not be used with thioridazine, an antipsychotic, because of the risk of significant ventricular arrhythmias and rapid death.

Alcohol:

Alcohol can aggravate the negative effects of dapoxetine, including dizziness, sleepiness, and reduced cognitive function, raising the risk of harm. Patients are recommended not to consume alcohol while using dapoxetine.

Central Nervous System (CNS) depressants:

Concurrent use of dapoxetine with CNS depressants such as opioids, benzodiazepines, and some antihistamines might exacerbate CNS depression, increasing drowsiness and the risk of an accident.

Warfarin and other anticoagulants:

Dapoxetine may interact with warfarin and other anticoagulants, influencing blood coagulation. When these drugs are administered simultaneously, it is suggested that coagulation parameters be monitored.

## CHAPTER EIGHT

What are the common side effects of Dapoxetine?

Dapoxetine, while beneficial for treating premature ejaculation

(PE), has a number of typical adverse effects. These adverse effects are usually mild to moderate in severity and tend to subside with continuing usage of the medicine. These are the most often reported adverse effects:

Nausea:

The most common negative effect observed with dapoxetine is nausea. It can happen soon after taking the drug and can be alleviated by taking it with food or changing the dose.

Dizziness:

Dizziness, particularly orthostatic hypotension (a dip in blood pressure while standing), is another common side effect. This might cause a feeling of lightheadedness or fainting, especially if the person stands up suddenly.

Headache:

Users of dapoxetine frequently report headaches. These can range from mild to moderate, and can be treated with over-the-counter pain medicines if needed.

Diarrhea:

Some people have diarrhea after taking dapoxetine. This adverse effect is often mild and temporary, although it can be irritating for some patients.

Insomnia:

Dapoxetine may cause difficulty sleeping or insomnia. This negative effect could be due to the medication's effects on the central nervous system.

Fatigue:

Fatigue or fatigue is another commonly mentioned adverse effect. It can affect everyday activities and overall energy levels, but it usually fades with continuing usage of the medicine.

Dry mouth.

Dry mouth is a typical side effect that can cause discomfort and heighten the risk of dental problems. Drinking plenty of water and using sugar-free gum or lozenges can assist with this symptom.

Sweating:

Some people who take dapoxetine have noticed increased sweating, particularly at night. This can be mitigated by staying hydrated and wearing breathable clothing.

Restlessness and anxiety:

Some people may experience more restlessness or anxiety. These symptoms can be controlled by lifestyle changes and, if necessary, consultation with a healthcare specialist for extra assistance.

Blurred vision:

Blurred vision, while uncommon, can occur and impair the ability to do duties that need clear vision, such as driving.

Ejaculatory Delay:

While dapoxetine is intended to delay ejaculation, it might cause abnormally protracted ejaculation or anorgasmia (difficulty achieving orgasm).

Palpitations:

Some people may suffer palpitations or the sensation of a speeding heart. This is usually moderate, but it should be monitored.

# CHAPTER NINE
## Key Takeaways regarding Dapoxetine

Dapoxetine is a drug primarily used for the treatment of premature ejaculation (PE), and it provides several major takeaways:

Dapoxetine acts as a selective serotonin reuptake inhibitor (SSRI), boosting serotonin levels in the brain. This improves control of ejaculation by delaying the ejaculatory response.

Onset and Duration: Unlike other SSRIs used to treat mood disorders, dapoxetine has a fast onset of action, usually within 1-3 hours of consumption. Its short half-life of about 1.5 hours enables on-demand use, making it ideal for males looking for fast improvement in ejaculatory control.

Dapoxetine is given orally in tablet form, often 1-3 hours before planned sexual activity. The recommended dosage ranges between 30 mg and 60 mg, with changes dependent on individual reaction and tolerance.

Effectiveness: Clinical investigations have demonstrated that dapoxetine increases intravaginal ejaculatory latency time (IELT) and improves ejaculatory control. It also increases sexual satisfaction while reducing the psychological pain associated with PE.

Dapoxetine's common adverse effects include nausea, dizziness, headache, diarrhea, and insomnia. These adverse effects are typically mild to moderate in severity and frequently subside with continuous use.

Contraindications: Dapoxetine is not recommended for people with serious cardiovascular diseases, severe hepatic impairment, or who are taking specific drugs (e.g., MAOIs, powerful CYP3A4 inhibitors) due to the risk of side effects or interactions.

Drug Interactions: Dapoxetine may interact with other drugs, especially those that influence serotonin levels or metabolism. When using dapoxetine in conjunction with other medications, careful evaluation and monitoring are required.

Side Effect Management: Managing dapoxetine side effects requires lifestyle changes such as dietary changes, proper hydration, excellent sleep hygiene, and, in certain cases, drug adjustments under medical supervision.

Patient Considerations: Before beginning dapoxetine treatment, individuals should have a full medical evaluation to determine suitability and discuss potential risks and benefits with a healthcare specialist.

Quality of Life: Dapoxetine is a well-tolerated and effective therapy choice for men with PE, greatly enhancing sexual function and overall quality of life.

Overall, dapoxetine is a targeted and beneficial therapy choice for treating premature ejaculation, giving quick relief and increasing sexual satisfaction for both affected individuals and their partners.

THE END

www.ingramcontent.com/pod-product-compliance
Lightning Source LLC
Chambersburg PA
CBHW072021230526
45479CB00008B/317